MCQs for Student Paramedics

Covering anatomy & physiology, pharmacology, medical
conditions, trauma & resuscitation.

By Christoph Schroth

Why multiple-choice-questions?

Multiple-choice questions are a quick way of testing your knowledge or discovering an area to improve in. This is a collection of 150 peer-reviewed questions suitable for student paramedics at any stage of their education, covering key areas of anatomy & physiology, pharmacology, medical conditions, trauma and resuscitation. The answers can be found at the end of each chapter.

Thank you for taking the time to read this book. Please also have a look at my author page on Amazon for other available titles. I would appreciate it if you would leave a review of this book. Ideas and suggestions are also always appreciated.

I sincerely hope you will enjoy it,

Christoph

Table of Contents

Anatomy & Physiology Questions

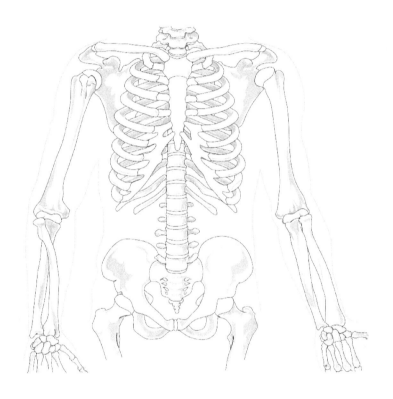

Question 1:
Cardiac output can be calculated using which formula?
   a) CO = HR x SV
   b) Q = HR x SV
   c) CO = HR x SV x SVR
   d) All of the above

Question 2:
Which one of these statements is true?
   a) Erythrocytes are red blood cells
   b) Leukocytes are white blood cells
   c) Platelets and thrombocytes are the same thing
   d) All of the above

Question 3:
Arterial pH should be:
   a) 7.31 – 7.41
   b) 7.35 – 7.45
   c) 7.45 – 7.55
   d) 7.25 – 7.55

Question 4:
Bell's palsy is a palsy of which cranial nerve?
   a) V – Trigeminal
   b) VI – Abducens
   c) VII – Facial
   d) VIII – Vestibulocochlear

Question 5:
The scaphoid is a:
   a) Metacarpal
   b) Carpal
   c) Metatarsal
   d) Tarsal

Question 6:
The 'lub' sound of the 'lub dub' heart sound is caused by what happening within the heart?
    a) The SA node depolarising
    b) Bicuspid and tricuspid valves closing
    c) Bicuspid and tricuspid valves opening
    d) Aortic and pulmonary valves closing

Question 7:
Which of these is not a response of the sympathetic nervous system?
    a) Nose glands produce more mucous
    b) Liver releases additional glucose
    c) Immune & reproductive system suppressed
    d) Increased sweating

Question 8:
Which parts of the brain form part of the limbic system? (Select all that apply)
    a) Cingulate cortex
    b) Hypothalamus
    c) Hippocampus
    d) Amygdala

Question 9:
Which tissue type is the body made up of?
    a) Connective tissue
    b) Nervous tissue
    c) Muscular tissue
    d) All of the above

Question 10:
Which of these are functions of the skin? (Select all that apply)
    a) Absorption & protection
    b) Sensory
    c) Vitamin D synthesis
    d) Excretion

Question 11:
Sphenoid, ethmoid, temporal & parietal are part of the:
   a) Skull
   b) Wrist
   c) Foot
   d) None of the above

Question 12:
Which of the following are part of the endocrine system?
   a) Glands
   b) Chemical messengers
   c) Islets of Langerhans
   d) All of the above

Question 13:
What is the correct order of the meninges, from the brain, outwards?
   a) Pia mater, dura mater, arachnoid mater
   b) Pia mater, arachnoid mater, dura mater
   c) Dura mater, arachnoid mater, pia mater
   d) Dura mater, pia mater, arachnoid mater

Question 14:
Which of these statements about zygotes is true?
   a) Once fertilised it develops into an embryo
   b) It begins its life as a single cell
   c) Its development involves two gametes
   d) All of the above are true

Question 15:
Which of these are types or components of bones? (Select all that apply)
   a) Sesamoid
   b) Osteoblast
   c) Haversian
   d) Periosteum

Question 16:
Telescoping of the bowel is referred to as:
   a) Intussusception
   b) Colitis
   c) Cholecystitis
   d) Diverticular disease

Question 17:
'Renal calculi' is commonly referred to as:
   a) Gallstones
   b) Constipation
   c) Kidney stones
   d) Crohn's disease

Question 18:
'Diffuse' pain in the abdomen would be:
   a) Epigastric pain
   b) Difficult to pinpoint
   c) Located at McBurney's point
   d) In the right iliac fossa

Question 19:
A significantly increased breathing rate can lead to:
   a) Hypercarbia
   b) Barocapnia
   c) Hypocapnia
   d) Acidosis

Question 20:
Laryngotracheobronchitis is commonly known as:
   a) Croup
   b) Epiglottitis
   c) Pneumonia
   d) Dysphagia

Question 21:
The coloured part of the eye is referred to as the:
    a) Cornea
    b) Pupil
    c) Iris
    d) Retina

Question 22:
The cerebellum is responsible for which of the following?
    a) Higher intellectual powers
    b) Smooth muscle control
    c) Sneezing
    d) Proprioception

Question 23:
Down syndrome is a trisomy of which chromosome?
    a) 20
    b) 21
    c) 22
    d) 23

Question 24:
The brain has how many ventricles?
    a) 1
    b) 5
    c) 4
    d) 2

Question 25:
The subscapularis belongs to which muscle group?
    a) Rotator cuff
    b) Quadriceps
    c) Triceps
    d) Pectoral

Answers

1 d
2 d
3 b
4 c
5 b
6 b
7 a
8 all
9 d
10 all
11 a
12 d
13 b
14 d
15 all
16 a
17 c
18 b
19 c
20 a
21 c
22 d
23 b
24 c
25 a

Pharmacology Questions

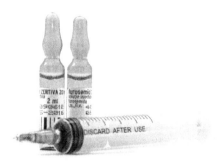

Question 26:
1mg of adrenaline in 10ml of sodium chloride (e.g. in a pre-filled syringe) equates to how many milligrams per millilitre?
   a) 0.1 mg/ml
   b) 0.01 mg/ml
   c) 1.0 mg/ml
   d) None of the above

Question 27:
What does half-life mean?
   a) The time it takes a drug to reach the liver or kidneys
   b) The time it takes a drug to reach half its original concentration in the bloodstream
   c) The time half-way between administration and peak plasma concentration
   d) The interval between repeat dosages

Question 28:
Midazolam may cause which of the following?
   a) Anxiety
   b) Hypotension
   c) Agitation/Aggression
   d) All of the above

Question 29:
What is bioavailability?
   a) How much of a drug is present after first-pass metabolism
   b) The average concentration of a drug in the bloodstream
   c) The percentage of an administered drug available in the bloodstream
   d) How much of a drug is available before being metabolised by the liver

Question 30:
Which of the following statements is correct?
a) Enteral medications are absorbed in the gastro-intestinal tract
b) Parenteral medications bypass the gastro-intestinal tract
c) Rectal and oral are both routes of enteral drug administration
d) All of the above are correct

Question 31:
Which mechanism would make glyceryl trinitrate spray and tablets largely ineffective, if they were swallowed, instead of being administered sublingually?
a) The therapeutic window effect
b) Coriolis effect
c) First-pass metabolism
d) All of the above

Question 32:
Subcutaneous injections are performed at what angle to the skin?
a) 15 degrees
b) 30 degrees
c) 45 degrees
d) 90 degrees

Question 33:
Which drugs are included for administration in an emergency under The Human Medicines Regulations 2012, Schedule 19?
a) Adrenaline 1:1000 (max. 1mg) in anaphylaxis
b) Atropine sulphate
c) Glucagon injection
d) All of the above

Question 34:
Tranexamic acid (TXA) is what type of pharmacological agent?
a) Fibrinolytic
b) Anti-fibrinolytic
c) Platelet aggregation inhibitor
d) All of the above

Question 35:
Carbamazepine, phenobarbital and phenytoin are all what types/class of drug?
a) Antipyretics
b) Alpha-agonists
c) Anticonvulsants
d) Anxiolytics

Question 36:
Which of the following statements about receptor stimulation are true?
a) Alpha 1 receptors – vasoconstriction & increase of blood pressure
b) Beta 1 receptors - increase of heart rate & strength of cardiac contraction
c) Beta 2 receptors - bronchodilation
d) All of the above

Question 37:
Which of these food products/supplements are likely to potentiate the effects of warfarin?
a) Garlic
b) Cumin
c) Cardamom
d) None of the above

Question 38:
An overdose with a tricyclic anti-depressant is likely to lead to which signs & symptoms?
a) Depressed level of consciousness
b) Hypotension & hypothermia
c) Seizures
d) All of the above

Question 39:
Which of the following suffixes of a generic medication name is most likely a beta-blocker?
a) -olol
b) -pril
c) -mycin
d) -zide

Question 40:
The mechanism of action of which drug does not involve cyclooxygenase (COX) enzymes?
a) Aspirin
b) Paracetamol
c) Chlorphenamine
d) All of the above

Question 41:
An oxygen cylinder left in a vehicle on a hot day would be affected by which law?
a) Henry's law
b) Charles' law
c) Boyle's law
d) None of the above

Question 42:
Drugs delivered via nebuliser to a pregnant patient will show results quicker than in a non-pregnant patient. True or false?

Question 43:
Which of the following is not a side-effect of prolonged steroid use?
  a) Increased intraocular pressure
  b) Decrease in bone density
  c) Gastric ulcers
  d) Immunosuppression

Question 44:
Furosemide is a:
  a) Loop diuretic
  b) Potassium sparing diuretic
  c) Thiazide diuretic
  d) None of the above

Question 45:
Beta-blockers can be described as which of the following?
  a) Positive chronotrope
  b) Negative chronotrope
  c) Positive inotrope
  d) Negative inotrope

Question 46:
Which of these weight conversions are incorrect?
  a) 1 stone = 6.35 kg
  b) 150 lbs = 68 kg
  c) 25kg = 6 stone
  d) All are incorrect

Question 47:
Which pharmacological abbreviation from medical records is incorrect?
  a) prn = as needed
  b) bid / bd = twice per day
  c) hs = at morning time
  d) od = once a day

Question 48:
To be the most effective, acetylcysteine should be given within
__ hours following a paracetamol overdose.
   a) 4 hours
   b) 6 hours
   c) 8 hours
   d) 10 hours

Question 49:
Possible side-effects of salbutamol include (select all that
apply):
   a) Headache
   b) Bradycardia
   c) Muscle cramps
   d) Rash

Question 50:
Hydroxocobalamin is indicated for patients with:
   a) Significant cyanide poisoning
   b) Ethylene glycol poisoning
   c) Heavy metal poisoning
   d) Carbon monoxide poisoning

Answers

26 a
27 b
28 d
29 c
30 d
31 c
32 c
33 d
34 b
35 c
36 d
37 a
38 d
39 a
40 c
41 b
42 True
43 a
44 a
45 b
46 c
47 c
48 c
49 all
50 a

Medical Questions

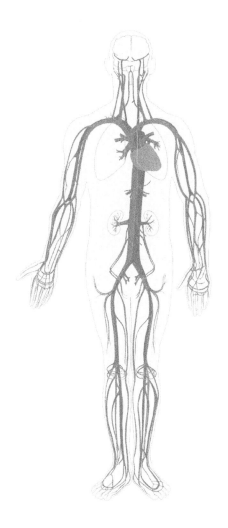

Question 51:
The NEWS2 (National Early Warning Score 2) assigns numerical scores to which of these physiological parameters?
   a) Respiratory rate & SpO2
   b) Systolic BP & pulse rate
   c) Level of consciousness or new onset confusion & temperature
   d) All of the above

Question 52:
Full dilation of the cervix until delivery of the baby is part of which stage/phase of labour?
   a) First stage
   b) Transitional phase
   c) Second stage
   d) Third stage

Question 53:
The Wells score (Wells Clinical Prediction Rule) is used to predict what?
   a) Likelihood of DVT (deep vein thrombosis)
   b) Severity of DVT
   c) CVA risk from DVT
   d) All of the above

Question 54:
Signs and symptoms of a TIA are identical to those of a CVA. True or false?

Question 55:
The ABCD2 scoring system assigns points to which of these areas?
   a) Age, BP, clinical features, duration of seizures, diabetes
   b) Age, blood glucose, clinical features, duration of symptoms, diabetes
   c) Age, BP, clinical features, duration of symptoms, diabetes
   d) None of the above

Question 56:
Which statement about Reye syndrome is not true?
a) It affects the liver and brain
b) Pupil responses are abnormal
c) Typically develops after a bacterial infection
d) May be associated with aspirin use

Question 57:
Which acronym can be used to remember the signs &
symptoms of organophosphate poisoning or cholinergic
overdoses?
a) PDDRTD
b) DUMBELLS
c) SLUDGE
d) B & C

Question 58:
Mean Arterial Pressure (MAP) is calculated by using which
formula?
a) MAP = Systolic BP + (2 x diastolic BP) / 3
b) MAP = Systolic BP + diastolic BP / 3
c) MAP = (2 x systolic BP) + diastolic BP / 4
d) MAP = (Systolic BP / diastolic) x 3

Question 59:
How much urine should an adult over the age of 65 years
produce per hour?
a) > 1.5 ml/kg/h
b) > 1 ml/kg/h
c) > 0.5 ml/kg/h
d) > 0.25 ml/kg/h

Question 60:
What is a key characteristic of String's sign on an ECG
(potential pointer towards hyperkalaemia)?
a) Flattened p-waves
b) Broadened QRS
c) Peaked T-waves
d) All of the above

Question 61:
Which acronym is most commonly used to assess pain?
a) SOCRATES
b) OPQRST(A)
c) AMPLE
d) A & B

Question 62:
Braxton-Hicks contractions are:
a) Non-uterine contractions
b) Uterine contractions
c) Generally painless
d) B & C

Question 63:
Which area does the FLACC scale include (to assess pain in children up to 7 years of age)?
a) Face & Legs
b) Activity, Cry & Consolability
c) A & B
d) None of the above

Question 64:
Indications for permanent pacing include:
a) Symptomatic 2nd degree heart block
b) Symptomatic bradycardia due to sick sinus syndrome
c) Symptomatic bradycardia due to atrioventricular block
d) All of the above

Question 65:
Signs & symptoms of pre-eclampsia include:
a) Vomiting
b) Visual problems
c) Severe headaches
d) All of the above

Question 66:
Which statement about Bell's palsy is false?
  a) It generally includes drooping of the eyelid/eyebrow
  b) It causes dilation of the pupil on the affected side
  c) It is usually caused by a virus
  d) Steroids may be used to treat it

Question 67:
A positive result when performing Murphy's sign would indicate which condition?
  a) Appendicitis
  b) Ectopic Pregnancy
  c) Gastric Ulcer
  d) Cholecystitis

Question 68:
Steatorrhoea is a sign of:
  a) Gastric ulcers
  b) Hepatitis
  c) Chronic pancreatic inflammation
  d) None of the above

Question 69:
When percussing a chest, hypo resonance is likely to have what cause?
  a) Increased air in the lungs
  b) Solid mass or fluid in the lungs
  c) Pneumothorax
  d) Pericarditis

Question 70:
In normal adult respiratory patterns, chest expansion should measure between:
  a) 6-7cm
  b) 4-5cm
  c) 10-11cm
  d) 7-8cm

Question 71:
Which 2 of these are systolic murmurs?
a) Aortic stenosis
b) Aortic regurgitation
c) Mitral stenosis
d) Mitral regurgitation

Question 72:
In a cardiovascular assessment, what are 'thrills'?
a) Different pulse rates at the carotid and radial sites
b) Palpable murmurs
c) Sustained impulse hitting the chest wall
d) An absent apical pulse

Question 73:
Hardened supraclavicular lymph nodes on the patients left side can indicate what?
a) Previous shoulder dislocation
b) Abdominal malignancy
c) The need for a breast scan in women
d) Brain tumour

Question 74:
The nodes referred to in the previous question are commonly referred to as:
a) Virchow's
b) Axillary
c) Sublingual
d) Paratracheal

Question 75:
Febrile convulsions commonly occur in children <5 years of age, due to a not yet fully developed:
a) Pituitary gland
b) Pancreas
c) Hypothalamus
d) Thyroid gland

Answers

51d
52 c
53 a
54 True
55 c
56 c
57 d
58 a
59 d
60 d
61 d
62 d
63 c
64 d
65 d
66 b
67 d
68 c
69 b
70 b
71 a & d
72 b
73 b
74 a
75 c

Trauma Questions

Question 76:
What is permissive hypotension?
- a) Restricting fluid resuscitation until haemorrhage is definitively controlled
- b) Only administering IV fluids until a 90mmHg systolic blood pressure is achieved
- c) Limiting IV fluid boluses to 250ml each
- d) All of the above

Question 77:
The landmarks for needle thoracentesis are (select all that apply):
- a) Mid-clavicular line in the 4th intercostal space
- b) Mid-clavicular line in the 2nd intercostal space
- c) Mid-axillary line in the 5th intercostal space
- d) Mix-axillary line in the 4th intercostal space

Question 78:
What are the three elements of the trauma triad / lethal triad?
- a) Acidosis, coagulopathy & hypotension
- b) Acidosis, coagulopathy & hypothermia
- c) Alkalosis, coagulopathy & hypotension
- d) Alkalosis, coagulopathy & hypothermia

Question 79:
Intracranial pressure in adults should be approximately:
- a) 2 – 10 mmHg
- b) 10 – 20 mmHg
- c) 6 – 18 mmHg
- d) 5 – 15 mmHg

Question 80:
Which of the following are signs & symptoms of a tension pneumothorax?
- a) Shortness of breath
- b) Decreased air entry on the affected side
- c) Hypo-resonance on percussion
- d) A & B

Question 81:
Jugular venous distension, trachea at the midline, normo-resonance on percussion & muffled heart sounds are most likely signs of a:
a) Pericardial tamponade
b) Tension pneumothorax
c) Pleural effusion
d) None of the above

Question 82:
The Rule of Nines (to estimate total burnt surface area) should include which degree/levels of burns? (Select all that apply)
a) Superficial burns
b) Partial thickness burns
c) Full thickness burns
d) All of the above

Question 83:
Pain when palpating the 'anatomical snuff box' could be indicative of what fracture?
a) Patella Fracture
b) Scaphoid Fracture
c) Clavicle Fracture
d) Malleolar Fracture

Question 84:
The coagulation cascade includes which elements?
a) Tissue factor VIIa
b) Plasmin
c) Thrombin
d) All of the above

Question 85:
Which statement about blast injuries is not true?
a) Primary injuries are due to the pressure wave from the explosion
b) Secondary injuries are due to flying debris
c) Tertiary injuries are due to the patient being thrown against a stationary object
d) All of these are correct

Question 86:
In which situation could a needle cricothyroidotomy be indicated? (Select all that apply)
a) Inability to intubate with or without a bougie
b) All other stepwise airway management options have failed
c) Trismus
d) Airway obstruction below the vocal cords

Question 87:
Wound glue may be suitable for lacerations involving the:
a) Nose
b) Joints
c) Eyebrow
d) Upper lip

Question 88:
How many litres of intravenous, crystalloid fluids is the equivalent of one litre of blood in the body?
a) 1 litre
b) 2 litres
c) 3 litres
d) 4 litres

Question 89:
According to NICE guidance, adults with a head injury require a CT head scan, if:
  a) They have vomited more than once
  b) They have a GCS below 15/15 upon initial assessment in the ED
  c) A & B
  d) None of the above

Question 90:
Blood loss from a femur fracture could be as high as:
  a) 250 – 500 ml
  b) 500 – 750 ml
  c) 750 – 1000 ml
  d) 1000 – 2000 ml

Question 91:
Cerebral perfusion pressure (CPP) is calculated using which formula?
  a) CPP = systolic BP – ICP
  b) CPP = MAP – ICP
  c) CPP = MAP – diastolic BP
  d) CPP = MAP – (systolic – diastolic BP)

Question 92:
Which spinal nerve innervates the diaphragm and controls the rate of breathing?
  a) Phrenic
  b) Vagus
  c) Sciatic
  d) Intercostal

Question 93:
Cushing's triad comprises of:
 a) Irregular respirations, bradycardia, narrowing pulse pressure
 b) Irregular respirations, tachycardia, widening pulse pressure
 c) Irregular respirations, bradycardia, widening pulse pressure
 d) None of the above

Question 94:
Paradoxical breathing is most likely to be seen in which condition?
 a) Open pneumothorax
 b) Flail chest
 c) Haemothorax
 d) All of the above

Question 95:
Which element is not part of Beck's triad?
 a) Hypotension
 b) JVD
 c) Muffled heart sounds
 d) Tachycardia

Question 96:
Signs & symptoms suggestive of a traumatic brain injury (TBI) include (select all that apply):
 a) CSF/blood coming from the nose/ears
 b) Nausea & vomiting
 c) Amnesia
 d) Posturing

Question 97:
A pelvic splint can be used to stabilise which type of fracture?
 a) Lateral compression fracture
 b) Anterior-posterior compression fracture
 c) Vertical shear
 d) All of the above

Question 98:
The appropriate medical terminology for 'Raccoon eyes' is:
  a) Periorbital ecchymosis
  b) Transorbital ecchymosis
  c) Eyelid ecchymosis
  d) Subconjunctival ecchymosis

Question 99:
Which of these statements about thermal burns is incorrect?
  a) Should be irrigated for 20 – 30 minutes
  b) Should be elevated to reduce risk of oedema
  c) Must always be referred to specialist care
  d) Cling film should be layered over the burnt area

Question 100:
The 'Deadly Dozen' of thoracic trauma includes which of the following (select all that apply):
  a) Tension pneumothorax
  b) Cardiac tamponade
  c) Flail chest
  d) Myocardial contusion

Answers

76 a
77 b & c
78 b
79 d
80 d
81 a
82 b & c
83 b
84 d
85 d
86 a & b & c
87 c
88 c
89 a
90 d
91 b
92 a
93 c
94 b
95 d
96 all
97 d
98 a
99 c
100 all

Resuscitation Questions

Question 101:
End-tidal carbon dioxide should be in what range? (Select all that apply)
   a) 35 – 45 mmHg
   b) 30 – 40 mmHg
   c) 3.6 – 6.0 kPa
   d) 4.2 – 7.1 kPa

Question 102:
Which statement about hypothermic patients in cardiac arrest, is true?
   a) Defibrillation energy and frequency need to be increased
   b) Defibrillation should be limited to three attempts, if core body temperature is under 30 degrees Celsius
   c) Adrenaline and amiodarone can be administered at the same intervals as in a normothermic patient
   d) Above 34 degrees Celsius drug therapy is the same as in normothermic patients

Question 103:
The recommended depth of an endotracheal tube in an adult, according to the UK Resuscitation Council (2015), is:
   a) 20 – 22 cm in males; 19 – 21 cm in females
   b) 22 – 23 cm in males; 20 – 22 cm in females
   c) 22 – 23 cm in males and females
   d) 22 – 23 cm in males; 21 – 22 cm in females

Question 104:
Defibrillation energy for paediatric patients should be delivered at what level?
   a) 2j/kg
   b) 4j/kg
   c) 6j/kg
   d) None of the above

Question 105:
Random, uncoordinated, electrical activity summarises which cardiac rhythm presentation?
   a) Ventricular fibrillation
   b) Atrial standstill
   c) Agonal rhythm
   d) Ventricular tachycardia

Question 106:
Intra-osseous access can be obtained at which anatomical landmarks? (Select all that apply)
   a) Sternum
   b) Proximal humerus
   c) Proximal tibia
   d) Distal tibia

Question 107:
The post-resuscitation care algorithm (2015) recommends what target temperature following ROSC?
   a) 32 – 36 degrees Celsius
   b) 34 – 36 degrees Celsius
   c) Normothermia
   d) Temperature recommendations are not given

Question 108:
According to the 2015 Resuscitation Council UK guidelines, the target blood glucose following ROSC should be:
   a) 4.0 mmol/L or higher
   b) 6.0 mmol/L or higher
   c) 8.0 mmol/L or less
   d) 10.0 mmol/L or less

Question 109:
Post-cardiac arrest syndrome includes which of the following?
   a) Brain injury
   b) Myocardial dysfunction
   c) Ischaemia/reperfusion response
   d) All of the above

Question 110:
Amiodarone (in cardiac arrest) is indicated for which presenting rhythms?
a) Ventricular fibrillation (refractory)
b) Pulseless ventricular tachycardia (refractory)
c) Pulseless electrical activity
d) A & B

Question 111:
Which of these conditions prevent organ donation after death?
a) Active cancer
b) Creutzfeldt-Jakob Disease
c) HIV & Hepatitis C (unless donated to someone suffering from the same disease)
d) All of the above

Question 112:
A blow to the anterior chest, resulting in ventricular fibrillation, is called:
a) Commotio cordis
b) Commotio retinae
c) Cardio corda
d) Cordis

Question 113:
What is the tidal volume per kilogram of an adult?
a) 3 – 5 ml/kg
b) 5 – 7 ml/kg
c) 7 – 9 ml/kg
d) None of the above

Question 114:
Resuscitation of a cardiac arrest from blunt trauma may be terminated under what conditions?
a) Unwitnessed cardiac arrest
b) Absence of organised, cardiac, electrical activity
c) No pupillary reflexes (on arrival)
d) All of the above

Question 115:
Transportation of patients with return of spontaneous circulation (ROSC) should be:
   a) Transported with their head elevated at 30 degrees (in the vehicle)
   b) Transported supine
   c) Carried feet first if going down any stairs
   d) All of the above

Question 116:
Absent breath sounds on the left side post endotracheal intubation indicates which of the following?
   a) Intubation of the right mainstem bronchus
   b) Leaking ET tube
   c) Obstruction in the larynx
   d) Oesophageal intubation

Question 117:
The weight of a paediatric patient (up to 10 years of age), can be calculated using which formula?
   a) Weight in kg = (Age/4) + 4
   b) Weight in kg = (Age + 4) x2
   c) Weight in kg = (Age + 6) x2
   d) None of the above

Question 118:
Which statement about basic life support in infants is correct? (Select all that apply)
   a) Compression to ventilation ratio is 15:2
   b) Compression depth should be one-third of the chest
   c) Chest compressions should be done with two fingers (if alone)
   d) The encircling thumb technique should be used with two responders present

Question 119:
When using an AED, adult pads and settings may be used on a paediatric patient, if no paediatric pads are available.
True or false?

Question 120:
With an advanced airway in place and no capnography data available, what ventilation rate is appropriate in an adult?
a) 6 – 8 breaths per minute
b) 8 – 10 breaths per minute
c) 12 – 14 breaths per minute
d) 14 – 16 breaths per minute

Question 121:
Chest compressions in a paediatric patient are indicated if:
a) The heart rate is <60 bpm despite sufficient oxygenation
b) after five rescue breaths there are no signs of life
c) All of the above
d) None of the above

Question 122:
Which of these is not a reversible cause in cardiac arrest?
a) a)Hypovolaemia
b) Hyperthermia
c) Thrombosis
d) Toxins

Question 123:
An apnoeic infant should be ventilated at what rate?
a) 20 – 30 breaths per minute
b) 15 – 35 breaths per minute
c) 30 – 40 breaths per minute
d) 25 – 50 breaths per minute

Question 124:
a) Which pulse point should be used in cardiac arrest in a patient <1 year of age?
a) Brachial
b) Carotid
c) Radial
d) All of the above

Question 125:
   a) 'Torsades de pointes' is a type of:
   a) Polymorphic ventricular tachycardia
   b) Monomorphic ventricular tachycardia
   c) Polymorphic atrial tachycardia
   d) Monomorphic atrial bradycardia

Answers

101 a & c
102 b
103 d
104 b
105 a
106 all
107 a
108 d
109 d
110 d
111 d
112 a
113 b
114 d
115 d
116 a
117 b
118 all
119 True
120 b
121 c
122 b
123 c
124 a
125 a

Mixed Questions

Question 126:
The MEND exam (for stroke) assesses which three areas?
   a) Mental status, extremities & neurological disabilities
   b) Mental status, cranial nerves & limbs
   c) Consciousness, cranial nerves & coordination
   d) Mental status, consciousness & limbs

Question 127:
Which of these is / are a tool to pre-alert a receiving facility?
   a) ATMIST
   b) ASHICE
   c) 9-line
   d) All of the above

Question 128:
Vincent's angina & Ludwig's angina both affect which part of the body?
   a) Heart
   b) Mouth
   c) Brain
   d) Abdomen

Question 129:
A patient opens his eyes to pain, is confused and localises pain; what is his GCS?
   a) 10/15
   b) 11/15
   c) 12/15
   d) 13/15

Question 130:
Kinetic energy is calculated with which formula?
   a) $KE = \frac{1}{2} mv^3$
   b) $KE = \frac{1}{2} mv^2$
   c) $KE = mv^2$
   d) $KE = 2 mv^2$

Question 131:
A patient is receiving oxygen at a FiO2 of 0.2; what is the percentage of oxygen being delivered / inspired?
a) 12%
b) 20%
c) 24%
d) None of the above

Question 132:
What are the five stages of grief (in order)?
a) Denial, anger, bargaining, depression, anxiety
b) Disbelief, aggression, bargaining, denial, anger
c) Denial, anger, bargaining, depression, acceptance
d) Disbelief, aggression, belief, denial, acceptance

Question 133:
The oxygen dissociation curve shows the relationship between which two items?
a) Oxygen and CO2
b) Oxygen saturation of haemoglobin and the partial pressure of oxygen
c) All of the above
d) None of the above

Question 134:
The TICLS acronym, generally used in the initial assessment of the appearance of paediatrics, contains which elements?
a) Look/Gaze and Speech/Cry
b) Tone & Interactiveness
c) Consolability
d) All of the above

Question 135:
The colon and the majority of the small intestine are located in which abdominal quadrant?
a) RUQ
b) LUQ
c) RLQ
d) LLQ

Question 136:
What is the maximum score on the APGAR scale?
- a) 12
- b) 10
- c) 9
- d) 8

Question 137:
The sweat gland is located in which layer of the skin?
- a) Epidermis
- b) Dermis
- c) Subcutaneous layer
- d) All of the above

Question 138:
H1N1 is also known as:
- a) Swine flu
- b) Influenza A
- c) Avian flu
- d) A & B

Question 139:
Which lobe of the brain is responsible for smell, speech and conscious thought?
- a) Frontal
- b) Occipital
- c) Parietal
- d) Temporal

Question 140:
Which of the following FiO2 (Fraction of inspired oxygen) values are correct?
- a) FiO2 of 0.2 = 20%
- b) FiO2 of 0.5 = 50%
- c) FiO2 of 1 = 100%
- d) All of the above

Question 141:
Boyle's Law states:
   a) Pressure and volume are inversely proportional
   b) Temperature and volume are directly proportional
   c) Pressure and volume are directly proportional
   d) Temperature and volume are inversely proportional

Question 142:
What is chronotropic incompetence?
   a) The inability of the heart to increase the rate due to increased oxygen demand
   b) The same as sinus node dysfunction
   c) The inability of the heart to increase its contractility
   d) None of the above

Question 143:
According to NICE guidance on lacerations, wounds greater than what length should preferably be closed with sutures?
   a) 4cm
   b) 5cm
   c) 6cm
   d) 7cm

Question 144:
Henry's Law states:
   a) The amount of gas dissolved in a liquid is equal to the partial pressures of the gases above the liquid
   b) $C = kP_{gas}$
   c) A & B
   d) None of the above

Question 145:
Pain when palpating McMurray's point is indicative of what illness?
   a) Appendicitis
   b) Cholecystitis
   c) Crohn's disease
   d) Diverticulitis

Question 146:
Drowning (according to the WHO, 2014) should only be categorised as:
a) Fatal or non-fatal
b) Wet or dry drowning
c) Primary or secondary drowning
d) All of the above

Question 147:
Contracting which of the following diseases does not result in lifelong immunity?
a) Measles
b) Mumps
c) Chickenpox
d) Hepatitis A

Question 148:
Decontamination at a CBRN incident takes place between which zones?
a) Hot zone & warm zone
b) Warm zone & cold zone
c) Cold zone & outside area
d) All of the above

Question 149:
A person who is unable to smell may be suffering from damage to which cranial nerve?
a) I – Olfactory
b) III – Oculomotor
c) VIII – Vestibulocochlear
d) XI – Accessory

Question 150:
What is endometriosis?
a) Endometrial tissue growing in the pelvic cavity
b) Ectopic pregnancy
c) Hypermenorrhoea
d) Hypomenorrhoea

Answers

126 b
127 d
128 b
129 b (E2, V4, M5)
130 b
131 b
132 c
133 b
134 d
135 d
136 b
137 b
138 d
139 a
140 d
141 a
142 a
143 b
144 c
145 a
146 a
147 c
148 b
149 a
150 a

Other books in this series

More titles of this book series will be released in the future. Please follow me on my Amazon author page to receive a notification. Thank you for your support.

Christoph

Printed in Great Britain
by Amazon

36327056R00036